AWAKENING AND HEALING WITH THE GOLDEN TEACHER

A Transformative Journey with Psilocybin

Vidya Shastry

DISCLAIMER

This book is intended as an informational and harm reduction resource only. It does not provide medical advice, diagnosis, or treatment. The content within is based on the author's personal research and experiences and should not be interpreted as professional recommendations or endorsements.

Psychedelic substances and herbal medicines mentioned in this book can have a range of risks and potential contraindications. It is crucial for readers to consult with a licensed physician or qualified healthcare provider before considering the use of any psychedelic substances or alternative therapies discussed herein. The reader is also encouraged to conduct further research and seek out multiple sources of information.

The author assumes no responsibility for any adverse effects or consequences that may arise from the use or application of the information contained in this book. The decision to engage with psychedelic therapy is deeply personal and should be approached with caution and informed consent.

This book is presented as one of many resources for those seeking to learn about trauma and explore alternative therapeutic approaches, including psychedelic therapy. The information provided is not a substitute for professional advice or treatment.

PREFACE

Welcome to *Awakening and Healing with The Golden Teacher*. In these pages, I invite you to join me on a profound voyage of transformation, healing, and self-discovery, facilitated by the remarkable power of psilocybin. This book offers a deeply personal account of my experiences with psychedelic therapy, shedding light on the broader implications for mental health and emotional well-being.

Over the course of three distinct sessions spread across two transformative years, I share my journey of overcoming deep-seated traumas and uncovering enlightenment under the gentle yet potent influence of the Golden Teacher. For much of my life, I masked my pain with work and routine, avoiding the confrontations necessary for genuine healing. This book chronicles my path from these self-imposed constraints to a place of profound personal freedom and clarity, allowing me to confront and ultimately heal from the past that haunted me.

The journey through long-buried and deeply lodged trauma is not merely about managing symptoms or finding temporary relief; it is about bravely unearthing the shadows that have long lingered in our subconscious. Trauma that has been festering for years, or even decades, can profoundly shape our day-to-day mental and emotional landscape, often manifesting in ways we may not fully understand. Psilocybin offers a unique and powerful tool for this deep inner work, providing a lens through which we can confront and process these buried experiences. This book emphasizes the importance of approaching this process with profound respect and care, acknowledging that while the path to healing can be intense and challenging, it also holds the potential for transformative breakthroughs.

For many who are uninitiated into the world of herbal medicine, the notion of using substances like psilocybin in therapeutic settings can seem unsettling and even daunting. The term "drugs" often evokes strong reactions, especially when they are not the regulated, state-approved pharmaceutical medications we are accustomed to. However, it is crucial to understand that psilocybin and other traditional psychedelics are now making significant strides in research-driven clinical trials. I have endeavored to explain the chemistry behind these substances, shedding light on their mechanisms and the emerging evidence of their therapeutic efficacy. As these substances transition from fringe to mainstream science, their potential for profound healing becomes increasingly apparent, challenging preconceived notions about what constitutes valid and effective therapy.

My aim is to demystify the therapeutic potential of psilocybin and to provide a heartfelt narrative that bridges personal experiences with a broader understanding of psychedelic therapy. Each chapter is crafted to preserve the emotional intensity of my journey, guiding you through new realms explored with intention and care. From preparation and session experiences to integration and practical guidance, this book serves as a comprehensive resource for anyone interested in the transformative power of psychedelic therapy.

However, it is essential to address the potential negative effects associated with any form of herbal medicine, including psilocybin. While the therapeutic potential is significant, misuse or unsupervised use of these substances can lead to psychological distress or adverse reactions (for example, "a bad trip" which can be very unsettling). Understanding these risks, alongside the outweighing benefits, is crucial. Educating yourself through this book, joining supportive groups, and seeking advice from qualified counselors and educators can help mitigate these risks and provide a clearer perspective on approaching psychedelic therapy safely and effectively with long-lasting results.

This book is the result of my personal journey, extensive study, and quest for information about psilocybin therapy for my history of childhood trauma which silently snowballed into my adult life. It reflects my experiences and the insights I have gained over many years. I urge you to conduct your own research and explore various resources before embarking on any psilocybin therapy. This approach will ensure a comprehensive understanding and a more informed decision-making process. I aim to provide an inclusive view of the historical context and current research surrounding psychedelics. Understanding these elements is crucial for anyone considering their therapeutic use. It is important to address common concerns, such as fears of addiction and dependence.

As you read, my sincere wish is that you find not just a story of personal growth but also a balanced view of the transformative potential of psychedelic therapy. May this book serve as both a guide and an inspiration whether you are a seeker on your own healing journey or self-discovery, a skeptic curious about the possibilities, or a practitioner exploring new dimensions of therapeutic techniques.

Welcome to my journey with *The Golden Teacher*.

A PREQUEL

In the midst of a life shaped by trauma, where relentless scars had taken their toll, I found myself stepping into the uncharted territory of psychedelic therapy. My journey did not begin with a sudden leap but rather through years of research and careful consideration. What followed was a series of profound sessions spread over two years, each one a portal into the depths of my mind, where I became both the canvas and the artist. Guided by a skilled therapist, I embarked on a transformative path that would radically alter my existence.

The purpose of this book is to illuminate psychedelic therapy as a viable alternative to conventional treatments for deep-seated trauma. In a world where material needs, societal roles, and obligations often overshadow personal well-being, trauma can fester, pushing us further into the abyss. Traditional approaches can sometimes fall short, masking symptoms rather than addressing the root causes of suffering.

Through my personal journey and the experiences of others, I aim to showcase the profound healing potential of psychedelics when used responsibly and ethically in a therapeutic context. This book will explore the historical and cultural roots of psychedelic use, the modern resurgence of interest, and the growing scientific evidence supporting their efficacy. It will provide practical guidance for those new to this path, ensuring that safety and ethical considerations remain paramount.

As someone who was once apprehensive and resistant, with a background in nursing and firsthand experience with addiction and mental illness, I offer an unbiased perspective on this alternative mode of healing. This book embraces the mind's innate capacity for self-discovery and transformation, offering a beacon of hope for those seeking deeper healing and a more profound understanding of themselves and the world around them.

INTRODUCTION: UNDERSTANDING TRAUMA

Trauma is an intense emotional response to a distressing event or series of events that overwhelms an individual's ability to cope. Imagine being in a situation where you feel utterly powerless, like being caught in a storm where every gust of wind feels like it's pushing you further away from safety. That's trauma - when something so intense shakes your very sense of self and leaves you grappling with feelings of fear, helplessness, or horror. It's not just about the event itself, but how deeply it affects your inner world, and in turn impacts daily activity.

There are several types of trauma. Acute trauma results from a single, overwhelming event such as an accident or natural disaster. Chronic trauma stems from repeated, prolonged exposure to distressing situations, like ongoing abuse or neglect. Complex trauma involves exposure to multiple, varied traumatic events, often within a relational context, such as growing up in an abusive household. Each type affects a person differently, but they all leave a mark on one's emotional and psychological state.

The impact of trauma can be profound and lasting, affecting individuals across their lifespan. In childhood, trauma can stunt emotional and cognitive development. Children may struggle with trust, struggle to regulate their emotions, or face difficulties in forming healthy relationships. Imagine a young child who, after experiencing a traumatic event, clings to their parents with a sense of fear, unable to feel safe even in familiar surroundings.

As adolescents, individuals might turn to risky behaviors or struggle with mental health issues like anxiety or depression. Their sense of self may be deeply shaken, leading to an internal conflict that feels like a raging storm inside them, obscuring their path to a stable identity and clear future.

In adulthood, trauma can manifest as persistent emotional pain, relationship issues, or difficulty with trust and intimacy. A person might feel like they're constantly walking through a fog, unable to fully connect with others or find joy in life. It's as if the trauma from the past casts a long shadow over their present, shaping how they interact with the world and themselves.

Even in older age, trauma can resurface or become more pronounced, particularly if the person is confronting the end of life or dealing with significant health changes. The unresolved wounds from the past may come back, sometimes feeling more acute as they reflect on their life's journey.

Understanding trauma involves recognizing the profound and often unseen impact it has on a person's emotional and psychological well-being. Trauma is not just a momentary event; it leaves a lasting imprint on the mind and body, influencing how individuals perceive themselves, others, and the world around them. It's essential to acknowledge that behind certain behaviors, emotional responses, and struggles lies a history of overwhelming experiences that may have shattered a person's sense of safety, trust, and self-worth.

Trauma can manifest in various ways, from anxiety, depression, and anger to more subtle signs such as difficulty in forming relationships, low self-esteem, or a persistent sense of fear and vulnerability. These manifestations are not weaknesses or failures on the part of the individual but rather adaptive responses to survive and cope with the unbearable.

Approaching trauma with empathy means understanding that healing is not a linear process, and that each person's journey is unique. It's about being present and non-judgmental, creating a safe space where individuals feel seen and heard. This involves a willingness to listen deeply, to validate their experiences, and to honor the complexity of their emotions without trying to fix or minimize them.

Offering support to those navigating the lingering effects of trauma requires patience and compassion. It involves helping them find pathways to healing, whether through therapy, creative expression, or building meaningful connections. It also means empowering them to reclaim their sense of self, to reconnect with their inner strength and resilience, and to rebuild their lives on their terms.

Ultimately, understanding trauma is about recognizing the courage it takes to confront and heal from past wounds. It's about supporting individuals as they transform their pain into growth, and as they move from a place of survival to one of thriving.

CHAPTER 1: UNDERSTANDING PSYCHEDELICS

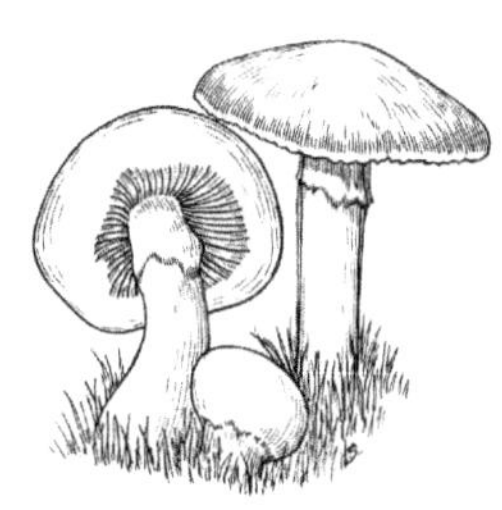

Psychedelic substances have long been revered in many traditional cultures, often viewed as sacred tools for spiritual and personal enlightenment. These naturally occurring compounds, such as psilocybin, LSD, and DMT, have been deliberately criminalized in modern societies, yet their profound potential for healing remains undeniable.

These substances, once held in high regard by indigenous cultures for their ability to connect individuals with the divine, are now being rediscovered by modern science for their therapeutic potential. They offer a unique pathway to healing, bridging the gap between ancient wisdom and contemporary mental health practices.

Psychedelics are substances that alter perception, mood, and cognitive processes. This chapter provides a foundational understanding of these compounds, detailing a few of their important chemical properties and effects on the brain. Let's explore commonly used psychedelics, explaining how they work and their unique characteristics. By demystifying these substances, readers gain insight into how psychedelics can facilitate profound psychological experiences, setting the stage for their application in therapy.

The Science and Wonders of Psychedelics

Imagine stepping into a world where your mind expands beyond its usual limits, where colours shimmer more brightly, emotions run deeper, and the boundaries of reality blur. This is the transformative potential of psychedelics - extraordinary substances that have captivated humans for centuries, offering a gateway to profound psychological experiences and personal growth.

In this chapter, we embark on a journey into the heart of psychedelics, revealing the scientific marvels and wondrous effects that make these substances so unique, unveiling the molecular magic that gives them their unique abilities, offering a foundational understanding of their chemistry and effects on the brain.

By interacting with serotonin receptors in the brain, these substances can induce altered states of consciousness, leading to experiences that range from vivid hallucinations to profound emotional insights. Let's explore the fascinating world of LSD, psilocybin, ayahuasca, and MDMA, uncovering how they work their magic in the brain and what sets each one apart, each with a unique story to tell.

We begin by delving into the chemical properties of some of the most well-known psychedelics: LSD, psilocybin, ayahuasca, and MDMA. This chapter embarks on a journey into the heart of these compounds.

LSD (Lysergic Acid Diethylamide)

Chemical formula: $C_{20}H_{25}N_3O$

LSD, often referred to as "acid," is a powerful hallucinogen that can transport you to the farthest reaches of your mind. Synthesized from ergotamine, a compound found in the ergot fungus, LSD's effects are like a kaleidoscope of sensory experiences. It interacts primarily with serotonin receptors in the brain, especially the 5-HT2A receptor, altering perception, mood, and cognition. Users often describe their trips as mind-bending journeys, with vivid visual distortions, enhanced colours, and a sense of interconnectedness with the universe, because it promotes heightened sensory experiences, profound introspective insights, and an altered sense of time, which can facilitate a deeper understanding of one's psyche.

Psilocybin

Chemical formula: $C_{12}H_{17}N_2O_4P$

Found in certain mushrooms, psilocybin is nature's guide; it gently opens the doors to mystical experiences, connecting users to a sense of oneness with the universe. Found in magic mushrooms (Psilocybe cubensis), it opens to mystical experiences. When ingested, psilocybin converts to psilocin, which binds to serotonin receptors and induces altered states of consciousness. This interaction leads to altered perception, mood, and cognition, allowing individuals to transcend their usual mental boundaries and confront deep-seated traumas with newfound clarity.

The experience can feel like a spiritual awakening, as users often report profound insights, emotional breakthroughs, and a deep sense of unity with nature. These "magic mushrooms" have been used for centuries in indigenous ceremonies, revered for their ability to open the mind to new dimensions of thought and feeling.

Ayahuasca

Chemical formula: $C_{12}H_{16}N_2$
Active ingredient is DMT (N,N-Dimethyltryptamine).

A traditional brew from the Amazon rainforest, ayahuasca is a potent concoction made from the Banisteriopsis caapi vine and the leaves of the Psychotria viridis plant. It is a powerful entheogen found in various plants and animals. Ayahuasca ceremonies are often guided by shamans who use the brew for healing and spiritual purposes. It is famed for its intense, visionary experiences and potential for deep psychological healing. Drinking ayahuasca can lead to intense, immersive visions, often described as journeys to and encounters with otherworldly realms. The experience can be profoundly cathartic, bringing deep-seated emotions and memories to the surface, paving the way for healing and transformation. DMT rapidly induces intense, immersive experiences that are often described as journeys to alternate dimensions or encounters with otherworldly beings.

Its mechanism involves binding to the serotonin receptors, particularly the 5-HT2A receptor, and rapidly altering consciousness.

MDMA (3,4-Methylenedioxymethamphetamine)

Chemical formula: $C_{11}H_{15}NO_2$

MDMA, commonly known as "ecstasy" or "molly," is celebrated for its unique ability to foster emotional openness and empathy making it particularly effective in trauma therapy. Unlike classic psychedelics, MDMA primarily enhances the release of serotonin, dopamine, and norepinephrine, creating feelings of euphoria, connectedness, and heightened sensory perception. It's particularly effective in therapeutic settings for treating trauma and PTSD, as it helps individuals access and process difficult emotions in a safe, supported environment. The warm, loving feelings it generates can make even the most challenging memories more approachable.

By demystifying these substances, we illuminate how psychedelics can facilitate profound psychological experiences. These compounds can unlock the subconscious, bringing repressed memories and emotions to the surface, and offering new perspectives on personal issues bringing repressed memories and emotions to the surface. This foundational knowledge sets the stage for understanding their transformative potential in therapeutic settings.

In summary, this chapter not only explains the science behind psychedelics but also reveals their wondrous capacity to open new pathways in the mind. By understanding how these substances work, readers can appreciate their power to facilitate deep psychological healing and growth, paving the way for their application in therapy.

In the realm of therapy and healing, psychedelics stand out as extraordinary substances that can reshape our perception, mood, and cognitive processes.

The Transformative Power of Psychedelics

Whether it's the deep introspection sparked by LSD, the spiritual awakening from psilocybin, the visionary journeys of ayahuasca, or the heart-opening effects of MDMA, each psychedelic offers a unique pathway to healing and self-discovery. My experiences have been with the psilocybin variety called the Golden Teacher.

Embracing the Journey

Understanding the science behind psychedelics is just the beginning. These substances invite us to explore the depths of our minds, challenge our perceptions, and embrace the unknown. For those curious about becoming users, it's essential to approach psychedelics with respect, awareness, and proper preparation. The set (your mindset) and setting (your environment) play crucial roles in shaping the experience. With the right guidance and intention, psychedelics can be powerful allies on the journey to self-awareness and emotional healing.

In summary, this chapter endeavours not only to explain the science behind psychedelics but also reveals their wondrous capacity to open new pathways in the mind. By understanding how these substances work, readers can appreciate their power to facilitate deep psychological healing and growth, paving the way for their application in therapy. Whether you're a seasoned psychonaut or a curious newcomer, the world of psychedelics awaits with the promise of transformation and enlightenment.

CHAPTER 2:
HISTORICAL CONTEXT
TO THE PRESENT

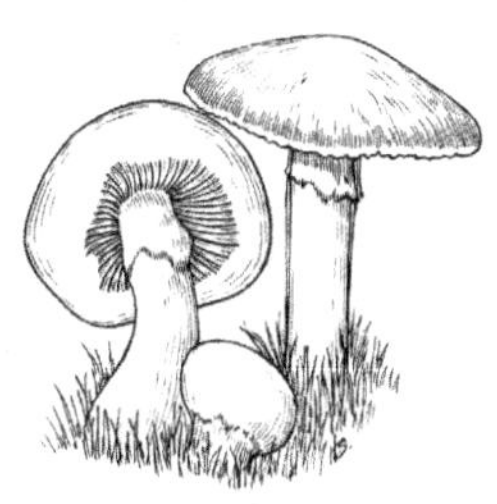

Psychedelics have a rich and varied history, deeply intertwined with the spiritual and healing practices of ancient and indigenous cultures. To the Western world, they are known from the shamanic rituals of the Americas to the Eleusinian Mysteries of ancient Greece, where they have learnt that these substances were revered as sacred tools for exploration of other realms and spiritual enlightenment.

This chapter traces the journey of psychedelic users from even earlier times in the Vedic Hindu rituals as mentioned in the treatise of ritual practices such as the Rigveda, to their popularization including the cultural impact in the 20th century, the upheaval of the 1960s due to this, the subsequent backlash during the War on Drugs, and the current psychedelic renaissance highlighting how renewed scientific interest is reshaping our understanding and acceptance of these substances in therapeutic settings.

Ancient and Indigenous Uses

The earliest known use of psychedelics dates back thousands of years. Indigenous cultures around the world have utilized plants and fungi with psychoactive properties in their spiritual and healing practices. For example, the Mazatec people of Mexico have long used psilocybin mushrooms in their ceremonies to communicate with the divine and to heal physical and psychological ailments. Similarly, the use of ayahuasca, a potent brew made from the *Banisteriopsis caapi* vine and other ingredients, has been central to the spiritual traditions of many Amazonian tribes. Psychedelics are also called entheogens or invokers of the divine.

Psychedelics, when used as entheogens, serve as powerful tools for inducing spiritual or mystical experiences that often lead to profound personal and spiritual insights. These substances have been utilized in various religious and shamanic traditions for centuries, facilitating deep connections with the divine or a higher consciousness. The term "entheogen" itself means "generating the divine within," highlighting the transformative potential of these substances in fostering a sense of interconnectedness, transcending the ego, and accessing altered states of awareness that can catalyze spiritual awakening and healing. In contemporary therapeutic settings, the entheogenic use of psychedelics continues to explore these spiritual dimensions, enhancing the therapeutic process and promoting holistic well-being.

Getting back to ancient Greece, the Eleusinian Mysteries, secretive religious rites held annually, are believed to have involved the consumption of a psychoactive potion called kykeon. Participants reported profound experiences of death and rebirth, suggesting a deep understanding of psychedelics' capacity to facilitate transformative spiritual experiences.

Recorded in the archaeological finds of Indus Valley in Northwestern India, Soma was a traditional brew used in rituals many thousand years ago in search of union with the Divine. It was an extract derived from Somalata, traced to a small shrub, *Ephedra gerardiana*, but there were many others in the original decoction. Even today, Som-ras is used as a potion/tonic but adulterated or the herbs substituted. A Wikipedia entry: "The ritual is not lost because of procedure but because of extinction of the plant. Some believe that soma rasa is not a single plant but a mixture of plant juices. Other scholars propose that the original Soma was the *Amanita muscari* mushroom, which is used by many shamans, particularly in Siberia." Ephedra from which ephedrine is derived is the source of many current day traditional medicines in India used for respiratory and cardiac conditions.

20th Century Popularization

The 20th century saw a renewed interest in psychedelics, beginning with the discovery of lysergic acid diethylamide (LSD) by Swiss chemist Albert Hofmann in 1938. Hofmann's serendipitous discovery of LSD's powerful effects in 1943 sparked a wave of scientific research. By the 1950s and 1960s, psychedelics like LSD and psilocybin were being studied for their potential therapeutic benefits, particularly in treating mental health conditions such as depression, anxiety, and addiction.

The 1960s also marked a cultural explosion of psychedelic use, fueled by the countercultural movement. Influential figures like Timothy Leary advocated for the use of psychedelics as tools for personal and societal transformation. This period saw the rise of iconic music, art, and literature that celebrated and reflected the psychedelic experience, leaving a lasting impact on popular culture.

The Backlash and War on Drugs

The widespread use of psychedelics during the 1960s eventually led to a political and societal backlash. Orchestrated fears of their impact on public health and social order culminated in the War on Drugs, initiated by President Richard Nixon in the early 1970s. All because of the failure to use it as a weapon to train soldiers to fight the enemy, which experiment instead made the soldiers see the true light of how connected humanity and Nature and all else was! There was no 'enemy'!

Not serving the experiment, psychedelics were then classified by the authorities in power as Schedule I substances, deemed to have no medical value and a high potential for abuse. This classification effectively and quite unceremoniously halted scientific research and stigmatized the use of these substances for decades.

The Psychedelic Renaissance

In recent years, however, there has been a resurgence of interest in psychedelics, often referred to as the psychedelic renaissance. Advances in neuroscience and psychology have reignited scientific curiosity, leading to a new wave of research exploring the therapeutic potential of substances like psilocybin, MDMA, and ayahuasca. Clinical trials have shown promising results, particularly in the treatment of PTSD, depression, anxiety, and addiction.

Organizations such as the Multidisciplinary Association for Psychedelic Studies (MAPS) and the Beckley Foundation have been at the forefront of this movement, advocating for the responsible and informed use of psychedelics in therapeutic settings. The growing body of evidence supporting the efficacy and safety of these substances is slowly reshaping public perception and policy, paving the way for their potential integration into mainstream medicine, just as advances in neuroscience has begun to reveal much of the neuroplasticity and 'rewiring' of the brain as with the advances of technology and tools to study the changes in the brain maps.

I have put in some names of books and journal articles for further reading at the end, however, there are many more resources out there in Google university and YouTube university - yours for the asking or googling! I have also appended a Glossary of terms used in this book which you can use as key words in the Search criteria when you are looking to exploring further. And for those who intend to be a user further exploration is mandated, in my opinion. Do not rush into the experience without good preparation nor just to have 'fun' with friends and acquaintances - as a recreational tool.

This is serious equipment to deal with a serious cause. Take it from me there are no bad trips; some dark corners that we would have intentionally or more likely, inadvertently repressed, being thrown up again. I'll soon give you some glimpses into how my therapist guided me on some of my very teary, sobbingly grief stricken persona, the traveller who was Myself but observed quite objectively by another Self.

The historical journey of psychedelics is a testament to their enduring significance and transformative potential. From ancient shamanic rituals to cutting-edge scientific research, these substances have continually been at the forefront of mankind's quest for healing and understanding. As we stand on the cusp of a new era in psychedelic therapy, it is crucial to honor this rich history and approach the future with an open mind and a commitment to evidence-based practice.

CHAPTER 3: THE HEALING POWER OF PSYCHEDELICS

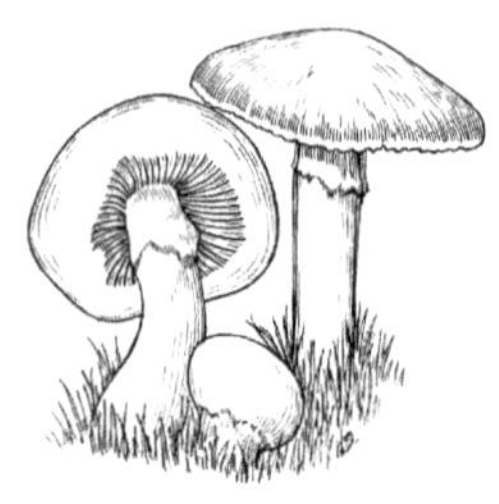

Modern research into psychedelics has opened up a world of hope, particularly for those struggling with mental health disorders. This chapter takes you on a journey through the key clinical studies and trials that reveal how psychedelics can be a beacon of light interacting with brain chemistry to produce therapeutic effects in treating conditions like depression, anxiety, PTSD, and addiction. We'll explore the science behind these findings, showing how these substances can work their magic on our brains. By the end, you'll see why psychedelics hold such promise and underscore the potential of psychedelics as powerful tools for mental health treatment.

Over the past decade, numerous clinical studies have provided compelling evidence for the therapeutic potential of psychedelics. Key findings in different areas of mental health include:

Depression: A Light in the Darkness

Imagine being trapped in a tunnel of darkness, with no end in sight. That's what depression feels like for many. But research at places like Johns Hopkins University and Imperial College London has shown that psilocybin can be a ray of hope. Participants in these studies, after receiving psilocybin, reported feeling lighter, happier, and more at peace. For some, these feelings lasted for weeks or even months. It's as if a heavy cloud lifted, revealing the sunshine they thought they'd never see again.

Anxiety: Finding Peace in the Storm

Anxiety, especially for those facing terminal illnesses, can feel like a relentless storm. But psilocybin has shown promise in calming these turbulent waters. In several studies, just one session with psilocybin helped patients find a sense of peace and acceptance. The relief they felt wasn't fleeting; it stayed with them, helping them navigate their end-of-life journey with a newfound purpose and tranquility.

Post Traumatic Stress Disorder (PTSD): Healing the Deep Wounds

PTSD is like carrying an invisible wound that never heals. But MDMA-assisted therapy has offered a path to healing. Clinical trials by the Multidisciplinary Association for Psychedelic Studies (MAPS) have shown that MDMA can significantly reduce PTSD symptoms. Some patients experienced such profound healing that they felt like their old selves again, free from the shadows of their traumatic past, experiencing complete remission after just a few sessions.

Addiction: Breaking Free from Chains

Addiction can feel like being trapped in unbreakable chains. But psychedelics like ibogaine and psilocybin have shown potential in breaking these chains.

Research indicates that these substances can offer deep psychological insights, helping individuals understand and overcome their addictions.
They also promote neuroplasticity, aiding in the formation of new, healthier habits. It's a glimpse of freedom that many thought they'd never see, aiding in forming new, healthier habits.

The Magic Behind the Science

The therapeutic effects of psychedelics come down to their interaction with our brain chemistry. These substances primarily affect the serotonin system, especially the 5-HT2A receptors, which are crucial for mood regulation and perception. By binding to these receptors, psychedelics enhance the release of neurotransmitters like glutamate, promoting synaptic plasticity - to form new neural connections - essentially helping the brain to rewire itself. Gone are the days when it was surmised that the neurons (and hence the brain as a whole) are set in number and function waiting only to be activated, but not allowed the luxury of rebuilding or resetting.

However, during a psychedelic experience, the brain undergoes significant changes:

Chemical Changes

Enhanced serotonin and glutamate activity lead

to increased synaptic plasticity, allowing for new neural connections to form. It's like giving your brain a chance to hit the reset button and start afresh.

Electrical Changes

Brain imaging studies have shown that psychedelics can disrupt the default mode network (DMN), one of the several brain networks associated with self-referential thoughts and the ego. This disruption can lead to a sense of interconnectedness and a reduction in rigid thought patterns that we have hitherto gotten to depend upon. It's a moment of clarity where you can see beyond your usual mental barriers.

Physical Changes

Long-term use of psychedelics, with curated doses and educated use, has been linked to increased dendritic growth and enhanced connectivity between different brain regions. This neuroplasticity or changes to the anatomy of the brain could be the key to lasting therapeutic benefits, helping the brain to stay healthy and resilient over time.

A New Dawn for Mental Health Treatment

The findings from modern research reveal the incredible potential of psychedelics as powerful tools for mental health treatment. By promoting neuroplasticity and facilitating profound psychological insights, psychedelics offer a novel approach to treating conditions that often resist conventional therapies.

As we continue to explore the therapeutic potential of these substances, it's crucial to ensure their use is grounded in rigorous scientific research and ethical clinical practices. This chapter highlights the transformative power of psychedelics, encouraging you to consider their role in the future of mental health care. Imagine a world where these ancient medicines are used to heal the mind and soul, offering hope and relief to those who need it the most in the current-day context.

CHAPTER 4: THE THERAPEUTIC PROCESS

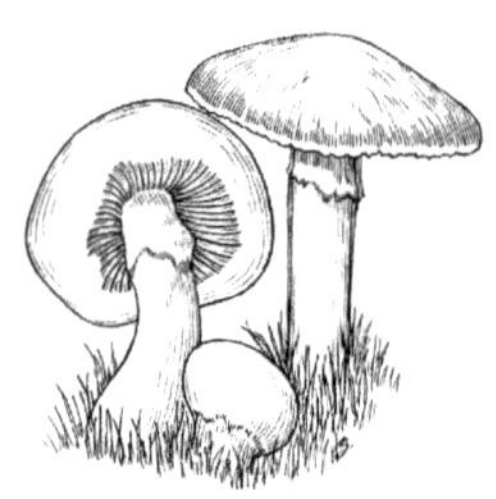

The therapeutic use of psychedelics involves careful preparation, guidance, and integration. This chapter outlines the stages of a psychedelic journey, emphasizing the importance of set and setting in shaping the experience. Let me discuss, in a few paragraphs, the critical role of therapists in providing support and ensuring safety, as well as techniques for integrating the insights gained from the psychedelic experience into everyday life. By understanding this process, readers gain clarity into how therapeutic psychedelic journeys are structured and facilitated.

Embarking on a psychedelic journey requires more than just the ingestion of a substance; it demands careful preparation, skilled guidance, and thoughtful integration. This chapter delves into the intricate process that transforms a psychedelic experience from a mere trip into a profound therapeutic journey, offering readers or listeners a glimpse into the meticulous planning and deep introspection that accompany this transformative path.

Setting the Stage

The foundation of a successful psychedelic journey lies in the concept of "set and setting." The "set" refers to the mindset of the individual - one's intentions, expectations, and emotional state, while the "setting" encompasses the physical and social environment in which the experience takes place. Both elements are crucial in shaping the nature and outcome of the journey. In preparation, I found myself delving deep into my intentions of confronting my fears and setting clear goals for what I hoped to uncover and heal. The setting was meticulously curated - a safe, comfortable space, often in the presence of my therapist-healer, who provided a grounding presence throughout the journey.

The Role of the Therapist

A therapist's role in psychedelic therapy cannot be overstated or undermined. They are the anchor in the storm, the guide through uncharted territories. My therapist was a beacon of support, helping me navigate the intense and often overwhelming emotions that surfaced. Coming from a long history dating back a couple of hundred years as she had thoroughly researched her ancestry, she is a passionate and compassionate helper in all ways. She ensured my safety, both physically and emotionally, and provided reassurance when I encountered the darkest corners of my psyche. The expertise she dealt with in recognizing and addressing the complex dynamics of trauma was instrumental in facilitating my healing process.

Techniques for Integration

Integration is the process of weaving the insights and revelations from the psychedelic experience into the fabric of everyday life. This stage is vital, as it allows for lasting change and growth. After each session, my therapist and I engaged in deep conversations, reflecting on the visions and emotions that had emerged. We employed various techniques, such as journaling, meditation, and somatic practices, to anchor these insights into my daily routine. This integration work was not just about understanding my past but about reshaping my present and future, creating new pathways of thought and behaviour that aligned with my newfound sense of self.

Preparing for the Journey

The preparation for a psychedelic journey is akin to preparing for a sacred ritual. It involves setting clear intentions, cultivating a mindset of openness and curiosity, and creating a supportive environment. This preparation phase is essential for maximizing the therapeutic potential of the experience. I spent weeks, sometimes months, getting ready for each session, engaging in mindfulness practices, and discussing my hopes and fears with my therapist. This preparatory work laid the groundwork for the deep healing that would follow. As you would expect, a lot of reading and researching into the topic went hand in hand.

By giving you a sneak peak into the therapeutic process, this chapter aims to provide a pretty comprehensive understanding of how psychedelic journeys are structured and facilitated. It is through this careful orchestration of set, setting, guidance, and integration that profound personal transformation becomes possible. As you read on, may you gain a deeper appreciation for the meticulous care and profound intentionality that underpin these extraordinary journeys into the depths of the human psyche.

CHAPTER 5: SUPERVISED VS. RECREATIONAL USE

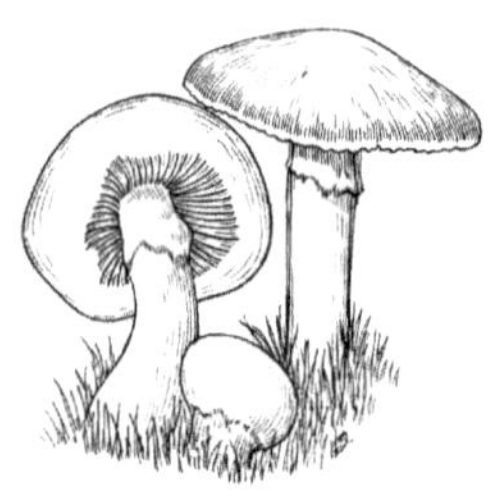

*Psychedelics, such as **psilocybin** (from certain mushrooms), **LSD** (lysergic acid diethylamide), and **MDMA** (3,4-methylenedioxymethamphetamine, sometimes referred to as "ecstasy"), all influence brain chemistry in unique ways that can affect perception, mood, and thought processes. Recreationally, these substances are often taken for their mood-enhancing and hallucinogenic properties in unsupervised environments, typically without structured guidance on dosage, setting, or intent. Conversely, in supervised therapeutic settings, the purpose, environment, and support are designed to promote safety and maximize psychological benefits.*

Supervised Therapeutic Use

In therapeutic contexts, psychedelics are administered under the care of trained professionals. A clear therapeutic intent, like addressing **treatment-resistant depression** or **post-traumatic stress disorder (PTSD)**, is established beforehand. During sessions, psychedelics are used to foster conditions that may promote **neuroplasticity**—the brain's ability to reorganize and form new connections, potentially allowing patients to "reprocess" traumatic memories or explore deeply ingrained emotional patterns with professional guidance.

Therapeutic use is tightly controlled to help mitigate the unpredictability of these experiences. Patients undergo thorough preparation, the environment is calming and supportive, and professionals are present to help the participant manage any intense feelings that may arise. In conditions like PTSD or severe depression, these substances may help break down mental "walls" created by trauma or emotional rigidity, opening new avenues for growth and healing.

Recreational Use

When used recreationally, psychedelics can indeed

evoke intense, life-altering experiences, but without guidance or a structured environment, outcomes are less predictable, or able to be correctly interpreted. Dosage levels may vary widely, and individuals often don't have access to support if the experience takes a negative turn. This is where terms like "bad trip" come in - a common issue when psychedelics are used without safeguards. **Psilocybin**, for example, can lead to euphoric, mystical experiences, but it may also lead to frightening hallucinations or paranoia if the user is anxious or unprepared for intense emotions. **MDMA**, often seen as a "party drug," can result in dehydration or heightened emotional vulnerability, which, without a safe setting, can lead to unintended consequences.

Additionally, the brain's **serotonergic system** (the neural pathways impacted by these substances) may be over- or under-stimulated depending on the specific substance and dosage. Unsupervised, this could lead to emotional distress, panic, or even psychological harm in the long term if users experience chronic anxiety or mood shifts after intense experiences.

Key Differences in Outcome

The main distinctions between recreational and supervised use lie in **intention, control, and support**. Supervised therapy seeks to build resilience, reframe trauma, and foster lasting positive changes. Recreational use, however, often lacks a therapeutic framework, which can leave participants feeling psychologically vulnerable or even traumatized by negative experiences, without resources for proper integration afterward.

To illustrate, consider that **psilocybin** in supervised settings has been shown to help rewire responses to negative stimuli through neuroplastic changes. Recreational users, however, may encounter uncontrolled or frightening hallucinatory experiences that lack therapeutic framing, leaving them with unresolved fears or anxieties. Likewise, **MDMA-assisted therapy** is a promising tool for enhancing trust and emotional openness in controlled, therapeutic interactions, but recreational use often prioritizes immediate euphoria over long-term emotional health, sometimes resulting in overstimulation or negative aftereffects.

Ultimately, supervised therapeutic use of psychedelics is designed to facilitate healing through controlled, purpose-driven exploration of consciousness, whereas recreational use can lead to unanticipated effects without the structure to process them meaningfully. As psychedelics gain recognition as therapeutic agents, understanding the importance of controlled settings, professional guidance, and clear therapeutic intent becomes essential to fully harness their potential benefits.

Let's delve into the nature of "bad trips" or unexpected reactions that can arise in unsupervised psychedelic use. These experiences often stem from the unpreparedness or inexperience of the user, combined with the inherent unpredictability of psychedelics. While they are known for their potential to induce euphoria and insight, they can just as easily lead to intense distress if used without the right knowledge, support, or setting.

The Anatomy of a "Bad Trip": Common Triggers and Effects

Lack of Emotional Preparation

Psychedelics like **psilocybin** and **LSD** tend to amplify whatever emotional state a person is experiencing at the time of ingestion. If a user is feeling anxious, fearful, or uncertain before taking the substance, these feelings can escalate to extreme levels. Unresolved personal issues or past traumas may also surface in unexpected ways. Without professional guidance to help process these intense emotions, a user may feel overwhelmed, leading to an unpleasant, even traumatic experience.

Setting and Environmental Influence

A major component of psychedelic experiences is the setting in which they occur. In uncontrolled environments - like crowded parties, public spaces, or unfamiliar locations - users are exposed to unpredictable sensory inputs, like loud noises, sudden movements, or unfamiliar people. These factors can contribute to sensory overload, leading to paranoia or intense fear, or grief. The lack of a safe, controlled setting may push users into states of confusion or panic, especially if the experience begins to feel "out of control."

Hallucinations and Disorientation

Psychedelics can cause powerful visual and auditory hallucinations, which may be beautiful in one context but terrifying in another. Unsupervised users might encounter distressing or surreal visions, from feeling as though they are seeing frightening creatures to experiencing intense distortions in their own perception of time and reality. **LSD**, in particular, can lead to prolonged, intense visuals that may create feelings of detachment from reality (often called "ego dissolution"), which can be deeply unsettling for someone who is unprepared. For example, users might feel they are "losing themselves" or fear they will be permanently changed.

Note: In a prepared and informed setting, both ego dissolution and a permanent change towards a spiritualistic and a vastly inclusive mind broadening sense of well being is experienced!

Paranoia and Psychosis-Like Symptoms

Some psychedelics, especially in higher doses, can induce psychosis-like symptoms. These might include feelings of intense paranoia, delusional thinking, or a sense of being in danger. For instance, **psilocybin** or **LSD** can bring about a sense of impending doom, causing the user to believe they are dying or going insane - what some call the "dying of the ego." In therapeutic contexts, a trained therapist can help guide the user through these emotions, but in recreational settings, people may feel trapped in an unending state of fear or dread, which can leave a lasting psychological impact, in a negative way.

Anxiety, Panic, and the "Loop Effect"

When feelings of anxiety or fear take hold, it's common for inexperienced users to fall into a cognitive loop, where they repeatedly cycle through the same distressing thoughts. This loop effect is common in **LSD** trips, where users may worry they are "stuck" in the altered state forever, feeling as though they cannot escape. Such repetitive thought cycles can intensify anxiety, creating a spiral of panic that becomes increasingly difficult to break.

Physical Reactions and Lack of Control Over the Body

Psychedelics often produce physical sensations like nausea, sweating, dizziness, or changes in body temperature. In a controlled setting, these effects are normalized and discussed ahead of time, helping users understand that they are part of the process. However, recreational users may interpret these physical symptoms as signs of physical danger, leading to further panic. For example, the stimulant effects of **MDMA** may cause sweating and dehydration, which, if not properly managed, can lead to serious health risks like overheating or electrolyte imbalances, especially in environments like dance parties or festivals.

Aftereffects and Residual Anxiety

Even after the primary effects of the substance wear off, the residual psychological impact of a bad experience can linger, a phenomenon known as **Hallucinogen Persisting Perception Disorder (HPPD)**. People might experience ongoing anxiety, flashbacks, or disturbing memories of their trip. For some, a particularly bad trip can leave them with persistent anxiety, depression, or a sense of existential dread, particularly if they don't have a support system or means of understanding and processing the experience afterward.

Minimizing Risk with Safe Practices

In therapeutic settings, professionals work to ensure the right conditions - mindset, setting, dosage, and support - to allow psychedelics to reveal their therapeutic potential while minimizing these risks. Recreationally, however, without such preparation, users face heightened risks of distress, negative psychological aftereffects, and even long-term anxiety or fear.

In short, a safe and intentional approach to psychedelics, ideally in a supervised context, is essential for accessing their benefits while minimizing potential harm. Uncontrolled, recreational experimentation can lead not only to deeply distressing moments but also to lasting mental health challenges, underscoring the need for care, respect, and support when exploring altered states of consciousness.

CHAPTER 6: THE POWER OF PERSONAL STORIES

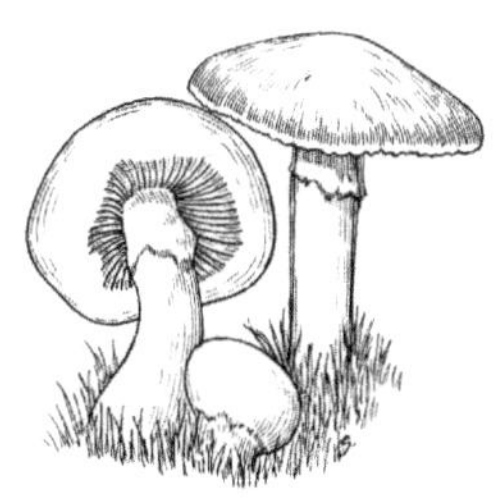

I offer these personal narratives to engage you with insightful moments to reflect upon. In the realm of therapeutic psychedelics, personal stories are the heart and soul. They are the whispered tales that speak directly to our innermost fears and hopes, the testimonies that ignite a spark within us. This chapter is dedicated to the significance of these narratives - how they can bolster your resolve and guide you if you choose to embark on your own psychedelic journey. Through the intertwining of instructional and personal elements, I aim to create a tapestry that could resonate deeply and inspire profoundly.

Personal Stories:
The Heartbeat of

Psychedelic Therapy

Personal stories are powerful tools for those considering a therapeutic psychedelic journey. They offer a window into the transformative potential of these experiences, providing reassurance and inspiration for those who may be uncertain or apprehensive. Each story contributes to a collective narrative that not only destigmatizes psychedelic therapy but also encourages others to explore their own paths of healing and growth. By sharing our experiences, we enrich the collective wisdom and compassion within the community, creating a tapestry of human experience that guides and supports others on their journeys.

These stories also serve as a crucial guide for those preparing for their own journeys. They offer lessons in self-compassion, resilience, and the importance of approaching the process with an open heart and mind. As you embark on your own path, let the experiences of those who have come before you inform your decisions, helping you embrace the unknown with curiosity and trust. Your journey will be unique, a deeply personal and transformative experience that will contribute to the broader narrative, illuminating the path for others and adding to the shared understanding of the healing power of psychedelics.

Embrace the unknown with curiosity, educate yourself as much as you can from as many resources as possible. Ask questions and find answers on the type of drug, the mechanism of its action, time tested and proven procedures; research the therapists, and then only trust in the process.

My experiences were always with psilocybin, *The Golden Teacher*, the gentle taskmaster who left no stone unturned as I delved deep into the labyrinths of my mind and soul. The medicine was in the form of a powder mixed into lemon-ginger tea spiked with natural honey to counter any unusual taste of the herb or onset of nausea. I was prepared by the therapist: I would take it on an empty stomach, and as the journey would last over an hour up to four hours, the honey would maintain the required blood sugar levels and my physical energy. I did not take any of my other medications before the session. Random blood glucose and vital sign (blood pressure and heart rate) readings assured me and the healer that I was well within healthy parameters at that time.

Initial Preparation and Expectations

Before the start of my very first psychedelic journey, I felt a mixture of excitement and a healthy

tension. My therapist and I discussed my goals: to address unresolved grief and the many traumatic experiences from my past, and to gain deeper self-understanding. I was hopeful yet apprehensive about what might surface during the session.
The anticipation was a mix of hope and fear, like standing on the edge of a diving board, knowing the plunge could be both terrifying and exhilarating.

Set and Setting

The session, in fact, all three sessions, took place in a cozy room with soft lighting and calming music. The music was optional and although I started with it, I soon turned it off and even wore noise-canceling headphones and an eye mask. The room itself was in a large, well-ventilated, and clean home in quiet and calm surroundings, with large windows opening onto mountains and water in the background, some island with lush green vegetation in the middle ground, and well-manicured lawns and a garden on which the house itself was sitting. The blinds were drawn. My therapist had arranged comfortable cushions and a blanket on the couch, creating a safe and nurturing environment. The atmosphere helped me feel grounded and supported as I prepared to embark on the journey. It felt like a warm, inviting cocoon where I could surrender to the experience without fear.

As advised, I had my journaling tools at hand: a writing pad and pen, and a glass of water if I felt thirsty. Before I drank the tea, I penned the purpose of my journey in my journal,with date and time, and what I hoped to achieve with this trip - to confront my deep-seated anxieties, although I didn't exactly know what they were.

The Onset of the Experience

As the substance began to take effect, I felt a gentle wave of warmth and anticipation wash over me, an exciting entry with a burst of colorful fireworks - dancing colors which became more and more vibrant, and my senses heightened. I had started the journey over which I had no control! All I felt was a sense of curiosity and openness to whatever might unfold. It was as if the world had taken on a new, magical quality, and I was seeing it through fresh eyes and wonder!

More and more sinuous plant-like objects unfolded ceaselessly, drawing me more and more into the interiors of the landscape, more and more endless paths, and a variety of bodies of water, small and large came into view from everywhere.

And they kept on welling up taking me deeper and deeper into an unending forest sometimes quite devoid of structures, many times with winding roads and hallways and staircases to negotiate and hills to climb, and valleys to descend into. I was exhilarated, as views and landscape changed constantly with a mix of buildings and woods. There was colourful vegetation that I did not recognize and labyrinthine buildings that were strangely familiar. Several emotions swept over me with great intensity. I found myself walking, running and even swimming and going against the tide. I walked endless miles. I waded through dark murky waters pushing aside huge blocks of a jigsaw puzzle of loosely arranged very huge Lego bricks.

Navigating the Psychedelic State

At the peak of the experience, I encountered vivid imagery and powerful emotions. I laughed, I cried, I sobbed. At times, I hyperventilated. My therapist heard me speak many times, and there was deep sadness and even intense grief in my expression and what I mumbled.

A multitude of faces flitted past me, and at one time a very ancient lady went past me. She was old, very old with white hair and a shawl, but she seemed fit and walked to her goal with a purpose. Images changed and sped past me with surprising alacrity and purposefulness. Landscapes changed with the speed of lightning.

At this point let me bring you back to my surroundings – at no time was I not aware of myself as a person. I knew who I was and where I was as soon as I opened my eyes. My healer encouraged me to step back and complete my journey. She asked a few questions, but I answered, only cryptically, she tells me later. I had voiced to her some traumatic events during my childhood, which we figured out in the debriefing sessions that followed later. I had seen a vision of a version of myself for whom I felt a deep sense of compassion. I saw family members, more than that I sensed them without seeing anyone. This realization brought a profound sense of understanding. It was like meeting an old friend I had forgotten. Was that me?

There were also moments of very intense joy that were so overwhelming, tears streamed down my cheeks, and I felt an awesome relief flooding over my entire being. I had never felt so much joy at one time ever in my life.

Each subsequent session had significant differences, and the differences had latent messages. One of the major perceptions was of gratitude. I felt immensely grateful, and I got down onto the floor. I wanted to be close to the earth. This is what I did during the last laps of my third and consolidation session. I walked into the garden and sat on the grass, close to the earth. My therapist sat with me. I was strangely quiet and pensive, she said. After the last session, I did not feel the need to talk. I had set my intention seeking clarity in the next phase of my life. I was extremely grateful and thankful for all my myriad blessings.

At one point, as I came out of the calm, quiet, and peaceful environs of the 'trance,' I said aloud to no one in particular – no one was in the room, anyway, 'So, what's the answer?' And a being, a… Being… It could even be me, whom I addressed later as 'You' in my journal, said very cryptically, "Now you know!"

That was it…?!!

My therapist debriefed me later. She says I had asked her to stay on and even held her hand during the initial part of the last session. To me, it felt like a few fleeting moments. Evidently, I had held on for over an hour!

The earlier trips had many distortions…furniture rising out to meet me, trees and shrubs in the pictures reaching out to me. When I had walked in the garden once, the grass shimmered in the sunlight, the plants reached out, and greeted me so lovingly, that later when I looked at the same shrubs, I said out loud, "How are you today, my friends?" The third consolidation session did not have any distortions. I saw the things around me as they were whenever I opened my eyes - it was into the second or third hour.

Another very impactful imagery I had on the second journey was of several bright and 'happy' entities surrounding me, and a very vivid act took place. There was a vibrant sun-like image and there were many tall evergreens and other trees and vegetation, bright colorful entity-buddies who surrounded me with joy and a great connectedness. I was engulfed by them all, and I in turn, engulfed them all as well! And this continued cyclically until we were all in a blissful, exhilarated state.

There was another very forceful and lucid moment: The mountain range yonder shook with mirth and laughed out heartily, telling me tales that I did not understand, but I joined in their celebration! Guffawing with wide grins, they shook all over, wishing me well and happiness in the future. They were like old friends with many tales to regale me with. and I was regaled, indeed!

Interactions with
the Therapist

During a particularly intense moment, my therapist guided me through deep breathing exercises and gentle reassurances. She spoke gently and calmly, but I was too far away to hear her. Her presence, however, helped me stay grounded and navigate the overwhelming emotions.

Emotional and Psychological Breakthroughs

At different parts of my journey, I experienced powerful emotional surges as I confronted overwhelming feelings of loss and grief. Tears flowed freely, and I felt a tremendous sense of relief. For the first time, I could fully acknowledge and accept these painful emotions, which had been buried for years, with ease. It was as if a dam had burst, and the flood of emotions carried away years of hidden pain. There was immense relief and lightness. I felt I could float away without a care in the world.

Challenging Moments: A Journey Through the Abyss of Re-emerging Trauma

Let me recount some of the details of my journey with a focus on the challenges that I wrestled with and emerged with some of the solutions for myself...

As I settled into the comforting nest of cushions and blankets, my therapist's calming presence reassured me that I was in a safe place. The room was dimly lit, with soft ambient music playing in the background, creating a sanctuary for the inner voyage I was about to undertake. With a deep breath, I ingested the psychedelic substance and closed my eyes, ready and willing to confront whatever lay hidden within the recesses of my mind.

The initial sensations were gentle - a warm, tingling wave of euphoria that washed over me, heightening my senses. Colours danced behind my closed eyelids, and a sense of boundless curiosity stirred within me. I felt myself slipping away from the ordinary world, descending into the depths of my consciousness.

As the journey progressed, I encountered a sudden shift. The vibrant colours and pleasant sensations gave way to a darker, more ominous presence. I found myself standing at the edge of a vast, shadowy abyss. The air around me grew heavy with an almost tangible weight of sorrow. My heart raced as a sense of intense dread took hold, and I hesitated, unsure if I could face it.

My therapist's voice broke through the growing tension, grounding me. "Stay with it," it gently encouraged. "You are safe. Allow yourself to explore what arises." And she resettled me on the couch, pulling the eye mask over my eyes and letting me sink back into the soft cushions.

With a deep breath, I stepped into the darkness. Almost immediately, I was engulfed by a torrent of emotions - grief, fear, and anguish swirled around me, forming a maelstrom of repressed memories.

Images from my past began to surface, each one more intense and vivid than the last, but they were not clear-cut scenes. It was more like I felt severe pangs of grief and loss that I had buried for so long. They erupted now like a volcano, its force overwhelming and sending my body somatically into racking sobs.

I felt the crushing weight of unprocessed grief pressing down on me, threatening to suffocate my very soul. Tears streamed down my face as I relived moments of profound sadness and despair. The scenes played out like a haunting film, each frame a reminder of wounds that had never truly healed. I saw the faces of loved ones or rather felt them, heard, no, experienced, the echoes of words that had cut deep, and felt the raw, unfiltered pain of those traumatic experiences. The re-emergence of traumatic life was experienced as a dark and intensely emotional grief experience during the journey.

Yet, amidst this storm of emotions, there was a strange sense of clarity. I realized that these re-emerging traumas were not just random flashes of my past but signposts guiding me to the core of my suffering. My therapist's presence, though unseen, felt like a lifeline, anchoring me as I navigated this emotional tempest.

In the heart of the abyss, I encountered a dark and

unsettling vision. I confronted the darkest parts of myself - the grief that had shaped my life in ways I had never fully understood. I allowed myself to feel the depth of my pain, to honour the tears that had been held back for so long. With each sob that racked my body, I felt a small piece of the burden lift.

As the journey continued, the darkness began to shift. The once terrifying abyss now seemed less menacing, its shadows less oppressive. I found myself standing on the other side, exhausted but lighter, as if a great weight had been lifted from my shoulders. The grief that had once felt insurmountable now seemed like a necessary part of my journey, no longer heavy and unwieldy.

Emerging from the depths, I opened my eyes and met my therapist's gaze. She led me into the garden to begin the process of integration. We discussed the intense emotions and vivid memories that had surfaced, and I felt a sense of catharsis - a release that had been long overdue.

In the days and weeks that followed, the insights from that dark and intensely emotional journey continued to unfold. I understood that facing my grief head-on had allowed me to reclaim parts of myself that had been lost to trauma. The re-emergence of these painful experiences, though harrowing, had ultimately led to profound healing and self-discovery.

Through this journey, I learned that true healing requires the courage to confront our deepest fears and the willingness to embrace the darkness within. It is through this process that we can emerge stronger, more whole, and more connected to our true selves.

During the integration process, I gradually realized that this darkness represented my repressed fears and insecurities. Confronting them head-on allowed me to transform these feelings into a sense of empowerment and resilience. It was a journey through my inner shadows, emerging stronger on the other side.

Integration and Reflection

After the final session, I felt a deep sense of calm and clarity. My therapist and I discussed the insights gained during the journeys. After, and at a rare moment or two during each session when I could write, I journaled my thoughts and emotions, capturing the profound realizations about my path forward. This process of reflection helped solidify the experience's impact on my psyche. It felt like stitching together the pieces of a quilt, creating a cohesive and beautiful narrative of my healing journey.

Long-Term Impact

In the months following the journey, I noticed significant changes in my emotional well-being. The unresolved grief I had carried for so long felt lighter, and I experienced a newfound sense of inner peace. The insights gained from the journey continued to inform my daily life, helping me approach challenges with greater self-awareness and compassion. It was like carrying a lantern within me, illuminating the path ahead with a gentle, guiding light. The path has not always been crystal clear; however, I can advise my cognitive brain to calm down and take a better look - reflect and make new sense of it. Many times, I felt on the verge of talking out loud, or making conversations, however, I suddenly did not feel the need to. There was a strange loss of peripheral noise, and my only focus was to look at the present and ground myself. I used many ways of grounding - I used my senses more keenly to look around me, hear and smell. I felt very calm and unrushed.

Why Personal Stories Matter

Personal stories like mine serve as a beacon of hope and understanding for those considering a therapeutic psychedelic journey. They provide a glimpse into the transformative potential of these experiences, offering reassurance and inspiration. By sharing our stories, we create a collective narrative that destigmatizes psychedelic therapy and encourages others to embark on their own paths of healing and growth. Each story adds a unique thread to the tapestry of human experience, enriching the collective wisdom and compassion we share.

Inspiring Your Journey

One key lesson from my psychedelic journey was the importance of self-compassion and letting go. Confronting my inner pain with kindness and understanding transformed my relationship with myself. I learned that healing is a continuous process, and each journey offers valuable insights that can guide personal growth.

CHAPTER 7: THE LEGAL LANDSCAPE

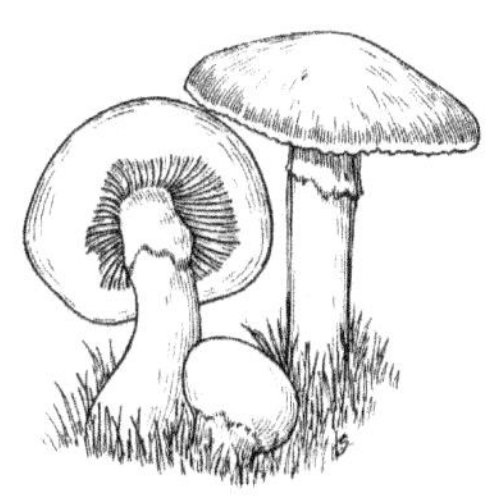

The evolving field of psychedelic therapy is marked by a complex interplay of legal and ethical considerations. As the therapeutic potential of psychedelics gains recognition, understanding the legal landscape and ethical imperatives becomes essential for practitioners and patients alike. This chapter delves into the current legal status of psychedelics, some recent changes and advocacy efforts, and the ethical framework necessary to ensure safe and responsible use.

The legal status of psychedelics varies significantly across different regions, creating a patchwork of regulations that can both hinder and facilitate their therapeutic use. In many countries, psychedelics like psilocybin, LSD, and MDMA are classified as Schedule I substances, indicating a high potential for abuse and no accepted medical use. This classification has historically stymied research and therapeutic applications.

However, recent developments signal a shift. In the United States, the Food and Drug Administration (FDA) has granted "Breakthrough Therapy" designation to psilocybin and MDMA, expediting their review for potential medical use. Cities such as Denver, Colorado, and Oakland, California, have decriminalized the possession and use of psilocybin mushrooms, and Oregon has passed Measure 109, allowing for the regulated therapeutic use of psilocybin. These changes reflect growing recognition of the therapeutic benefits of psychedelics and a move towards more lenient legal frameworks yet erring on the side of caution to ensure prevention of abuse.

Globally, countries like Canada, the Netherlands, and Portugal have adopted progressive stances, either decriminalizing or providing legal avenues for psychedelic therapy. These changes often stem from a combination of scientific advocacy, public support, and a re-evaluation of the War on Drugs' efficacy.

Advocacy Efforts and Legalization Movements

Advocacy plays a crucial role in shaping the legal

landscape of psychedelics. Organizations such as the Multidisciplinary Association for Psychedelic Studies (MAPS), the Beckley Foundation, and the Psychedelic Science Funders Collaborative are at the forefront of promoting research and policy reform. These groups work to educate policymakers, fund clinical trials, and mobilize public support.

Recent advocacy efforts have focused on a number of venues.

Public Education: Increasing Awareness and Safety Profile

Public education is a critical component of the advocacy efforts aimed at reforming psychedelic laws and promoting their therapeutic use. Effective public education involves disseminating accurate, evidence-based information to combat stigma, correct misconceptions, and highlight the benefits and safety of psychedelics. This book is also an attempt to lay out the foundational knowledge to a potential user as well as educate a recreational user who could understand the mechanism of action of these potent medicines. Better and become an informed consumer. Here are several key aspects of public education in this context:

Combating Stigma and Misconceptions

Psychedelics have long been stigmatized due

to their association with the counterculture movements of the 1960s and their classification as illegal substances. This stigma has contributed to widespread misconceptions about their safety and therapeutic potential. Public education aims to demystify psychedelics by providing clear, facts and information about what psychedelics are, how they work, and their potential therapeutic benefits, in varying degrees of participation. This also helps prevent misuse, abuse or unintentional disrespect for their therapeutic potential.

Highlight Historical and Cultural Context

Educate the public about the historical use of psychedelics in various cultures for healing and spiritual purposes, countering the narrative that they are solely recreational drugs.

Address Fear and Misinformation

Counteract sensationalized media portrayals and misinformation by presenting data from reputable scientific studies and clinical trials.

Promoting Scientific Research and Clinical Evidence

One of the most effective ways to change public perception is by showcasing robust scientific research and clinical evidence supporting the therapeutic use of psychedelics. Public education efforts can focus on:

Highlighting Clinical Trials

Share results from clinical trials demonstrating the efficacy of psychedelics in treating conditions such as PTSD, depression, anxiety, and substance use disorders.

Featuring Expert Opinions

Amplify the voices of respected scientists, clinicians, and researchers who can speak to the safety and therapeutic potential of psychedelics.

Providing Accessible Resources

Create and distribute easy-to-understand materials, such as brochures, websites, and videos, that explain the science behind psychedelics and their therapeutic effects.

Engaging with Media and Public Forums

Media plays a crucial role in shaping public opinion. Engaging with various media platforms and public forums can help reach a broader audience. Strategies include:

Leveraging Social Media

Utilize social media platforms to share educational content, success stories, and updates on psychedelic research and policy changes.

Participating in Public Events

Organize and participate in conferences, webinars, and community events to discuss the benefits of psychedelic therapy and answer questions from the public.

Collaborating with Influencers

Partner with influencers, celebrities, and thought leaders who can help spread the message and reach diverse audiences.

Empowering Patients and Advocates

Empowering individuals who have benefited from psychedelic therapy to share their stories can be a powerful tool in public education.

This involves a couple of platforms.

Patient Testimonials

Encourage patients who have experienced positive outcomes from psychedelic therapy to share their stories through videos, blogs, and public speaking engagements.

Advocate Training

Provide training and resources for advocates to effectively communicate the benefits and safety of psychedelics, helping to build a grassroots movement for change.

Educational Programs and Curriculum Development

Developing formal educational programs and integrating psychedelic education into existing curricula can foster a deeper understanding of these substances, which can include:

University Courses

Collaborate with academic institutions to develop courses and programs focused on psychedelic science, therapy, and policy.

Professional Training

Offer workshops and training programs for healthcare professionals to educate them about the potential benefits and ethical considerations of psychedelic therapy.

Public Workshops

Host workshops and seminars for the general public to provide comprehensive education on psychedelics.

Collaborating with Health Organizations

Partnerships with health organizations can lend credibility and reach to public education efforts. Working with these organizations can help in a number of ways.

Endorsement and Support

Seek endorsements from reputable health organizations to enhance the legitimacy of psychedelic education efforts.

Joint Campaigns

Collaborate on public health campaigns to raise awareness about the therapeutic potential and safety of psychedelics.

In summation, public education is vital in transforming the perception of psychedelics from illicit drugs to valuable therapeutic tools. By combating stigma, promoting scientific research, engaging with media, empowering patients, developing educational programs, and collaborating with health organizations, advocates can build a well-informed public that supports the integration of psychedelics into modern therapeutic practices.

Research Funding

Securing financial support for clinical trials to provide robust evidence for the efficacy of psychedelic-assisted therapy.

Policy Reform

Lobbying for changes in drug policy to facilitate research and clinical use of psychedelics.

Notable successes include the inclusion of MDMA-assisted therapy for PTSD in Phase 3 clinical trials, which, if successful, could lead to FDA approval. Such milestones are pivotal in transitioning psychedelics from illicit substances to recognized therapeutic agents.

Ethical Considerations in Psychedelic Therapy

The ethical considerations in psychedelic therapy are multifaceted, encompassing informed consent, safety protocols, and the potential for abuse. Ensuring that these ethical imperatives are met is crucial for the integrity and success of psychedelic therapy.

Informed Consent

Informed consent is a cornerstone of ethical psychedelic therapy. Patients must be fully aware of the potential risks, benefits, and uncertainties associated with psychedelic treatment. This involves a thorough explanation of the therapy process, possible side effects, and the experimental nature of many psychedelic treatments.

Safety Protocols

Safety protocols are essential to mitigate risks and ensure a supportive therapeutic environment. These protocols include a number of measures, the most important one being the very initial screening. Thorough screening of patients to identify any contraindications, such as a history of psychosis or certain medical conditions. The next is 'mind set' and the therapeutic environment.

Set and Setting

Emphasizing the importance of the set, the mental state of the patient, and the immediate milieu can significantly influence the therapeutic outcome.

Supervision

Ensuring that qualified professionals are present to guide and support patients throughout their psychedelic experience is essential especially for the first time user.

Potential for Abuse

The potential for abuse and dependency, though

very much lower compared to substances like opioids, remains a concern. Ethical psychedelic therapy must include safeguards to prevent misuse, such as the following aspects.

Regulated Dosing

Carefully controlled dosages administered in a clinical setting with emergency provisions, both to counter side effects (such as nausea or even vomiting) and providing first aid measures immediately at the onset of a journey, or later, as needed are crucially important. Mind you, a trained and an intuitive therapist will educate, prepare and initiate the participant with all the necessary information and wherewithal.

Ongoing Monitoring

Continuous assessment of patients to detect any signs of misuse or psychological distress, in future, is just as crucial. At the least, a few follow up sessions and debriefing are an integral part of an initial treatment, and most likely a suite of three or more journeys to consolidation. And settling down after the final session might, in all likelihood, take a few weeks to a few months. This is because of the 'rewiring' that takes place in the neuroplastic brain. The more informed or educated the participant is and their set and setting properly aligned, the better the integration proceeds to take place with effective results that one set out to obtain.

In sum, navigating the legal and ethical considerations of psychedelic therapy is a dynamic and evolving process. As research advances and public perception shifts, the legal framework surrounding psychedelics is likely to become more accommodating. However, ensuring that ethical standards are upheld is paramount to the safe and effective use of these powerful substances. Practitioners and participants must remain informed and vigilant as they navigate this promising but complex field, contributing to a future where psychedelic therapy is both legally accessible and ethically sound.

Legal and Ethical Considerations

The legal status of psychedelics varies worldwide, presenting challenges and opportunities for their therapeutic use. This chapter has explored the current legal landscape, including recent changes and ongoing advocacy efforts for legalization and decriminalization. We also addressed ethical considerations in psychedelic therapy, such as informed consent, safety protocols, and the potential for abuse. Understanding these legal and ethical issues is crucial for practitioners and participants navigating the evolving field of psychedelic therapy.

CHAPTER 8: CLIENT-CENTRIC PERSPECTIVES

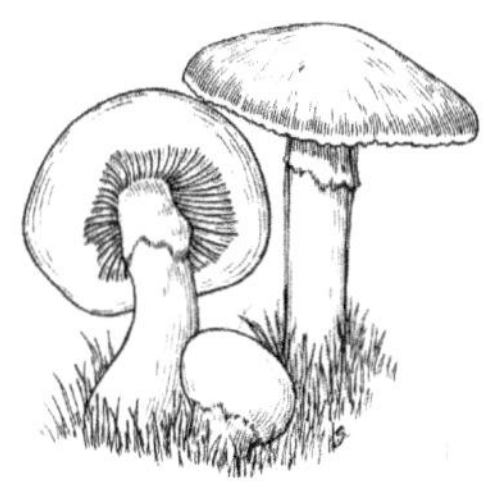

This chapter shifts focus from the therapist's view to that of the client or first-time participant. By delving into personal experiences, safety protocols, and therapeutic processes, the aim is to provide you with a comprehensive understanding of what to expect during psychedelic or herbal medicine therapy.

Psychedelics, such as psilocybin, ayahuasca, and MDMA, have shown promise in facilitating deep emotional release and processing of repressed trauma. They have garnered significant interest as a potential therapeutic tool as substances that can open pathways to the unconscious mind, allowing clients to access and work through repressed memories and emotions. However, their powerful effects necessitate careful and informed application within a therapeutic context.

Understanding the Client's Journey

Preparing for the Experience: Initial Consultation

Clients typically begin with an in-depth consultation to discuss their mental health history, current psychological state, and personal goals for therapy. This stage ensures that clients are suitable candidates for psychedelic therapy and helps establish a rapport with their therapist.

Before proceeding, clients receive detailed information about the potential benefits, risks, and uncertainties they may associate with psychedelic therapy. This transparency ensures they can make an informed decision about their participation and consent.

Clients are guided to set clear, meaningful intentions for their journey. These intentions help focus the therapeutic experience and provide a sense of direction during the session. Participants are encouraged to have journaling tools a hand.

Creating a safe space for a comfortable therapeutic environment is crucial. Therapists who pay attention to lighting, sound, and the presence of comforting objects to create a space where clients feel secure and supported make for good healers.

Building trust with the participant involves a strong therapeutic alliance characterized by empathy, and non-judgmental support. Clients need to feel understood and respected to open up during their sessions.

The Psychedelic Session: Guided Exploration

Entering the Experience

A therapeutic environment that feels safe and supportive for the client includes physical comfort as well as emotional safety, ensuring that the client feels secure and understood.
Gentle and non-intrusive techniques to guide the client through their journey, respecting their pace and boundaries and trauma-informed care emphasizes the importance of avoiding re-traumatization.

Clients begin their journey under the watchful guidance of their therapist. The therapist's role is to provide gentle support, encouraging clients to explore their inner experiences while ensuring their safety. Navigating emotions during the session is an important objective in a psychedelic journey.

Clients encounter repressed memories and emotions many times without any control over the wafting and even flooding waves of turbulent emotions that could be very somatic at times. The therapist helps them navigate these experiences, providing reassurance and grounding techniques as needed, their trained eye recognizing the swells, dips and calm plateaus in the traveller's inner journey offering help or words only when needed. It is a personal journey, and interruptions are minimal to only ensure safety to the traveller.

Post-Session Integration: Processing Insights

After the session, clients participate in debriefing sessions as integration meetings to process and make sense of their experiences. This step is vital for translating the insights gained into meaningful, lasting change.

Continued Support

Clients often engage in robust integration protocols of follow-up sessions, journaling, creative expression, and are encouraged to join support groups. Implementing them helps clients process to further integrate their experiences into their daily lives.

Ensuring Safety and Ethical Practices

Comprehensive Screening and Personalized Treatment Plans

A thorough mental health assessment is conducted to screen for contraindications such as a history of psychosis or certain medical conditions or use of medications, and medical and social history. This step is crucial for ensuring the client's safety, as well as educating them. Therapists tailor the therapy to the unique needs and circumstances of each client, ensuring a personalized approach that addresses their specific therapeutic goals, creating a supportive environment that can harness the potential of these powerful substances in an ethical and effective manner, while prioritizing the client's well-being and autonomy.

A flexible therapeutic approach of adapting the therapy based on the client's evolving needs and responses to the therapy ensures that the treatment remains relevant and effective.

Ethical Considerations

Psychoeducation

Clients are educated about the nature of psychedelics, their effects, and the therapeutic process. This helps in setting realistic expectations and reducing anxiety. Comprehensive and thorough preparation sessions that educate the client about the psychedelic experience address any fears or misconceptions and help them establish clear intentions for the therapy.

Informed Consent

Clients are continually informed about their therapy, including any new information or changes in the therapeutic plan. This ongoing process ensures they remain fully aware, more than adequately educated and consenting participants.

Confidentiality

Strict confidentiality is maintained regarding the client's participation in psychedelic therapy and their experiences during sessions, ensuring their privacy and trust.

Professional Boundaries

Therapists adhere to professional boundaries and ethical guidelines, focusing on the client's welfare and avoiding dual relationships. Real-time adjustments during the session based on the client's reactions and comfort level are to be made. This responsiveness helps to maintain a supportive and effective therapeutic environment.

Ethical and cultural sensitivity of the therapist are two most important aspects that a participant can look for during the intake process.

Acknowledging and respecting the client's cultural background and beliefs, incorporating culturally sensitive practices and considering the client's cultural context in the therapeutic process are as important as adhering to ethical guidelines and principles, ensuring that the client's dignity, rights, and well-being are upheld throughout the therapeutic process.

Personal Reflections

Empowering Experiences

Finding Clarity

Establishing a clear collaborative therapeutic relationship means clients take an active role in their healing process and are empowered to validate their experience and their autonomy is supported in making therapeutic decisions fostering mutual respect, recognizing the client as an expert in their own life and experiences.

Many clients report experiencing profound clarity during their sessions, gaining new perspectives on their past and present. This clarity often leads to significant emotional release and healing.

Emotional Release

Clients frequently describe the experience as deeply

cathartic, allowing them to process and release long-held traumas and repressed emotions.

Ongoing Transformation

Sustained Growth

The insights gained during psychedelic therapy often lead to sustained personal growth and transformation. Clients report improved mental health, better relationships, and a deeper understanding of themselves.

Community and Support

Engaging with support networks, including family, friends, and peer support groups, provides clients with additional emotional support and validation, helping them integrate their experiences more effectively.

These practices reflect the latest advancements and insights from researchers and counselors in the field, contributing to a more effective, transformative and most essentially a compassionate psychedelic therapy.

CHAPTER 9: SOCIETAL IMPLICATIONS

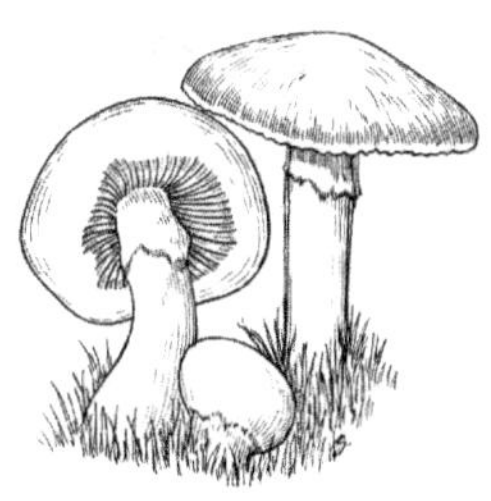

The therapeutic use of psychedelics is not just a personal journey; it's a societal one, with profound implications that ripple through our collective consciousness. This chapter delves into how these substances have the potential to foster spiritual growth, community healing, and a revolution in mental health care.

Awakening a Compassionate Society

Imagine a world where each person carries within them a spark of profound wisdom and compassion, ignited by their experiences with psychedelics. These substances have the power to guide individuals on deep spiritual journeys, revealing the interconnectedness of all life. When more people embrace this sense of unity, it naturally fosters a society rooted in empathy and understanding. Psychedelics can help individuals transcend their personal struggles, leading to insights that foster kindness and a deeper commitment to the well-being of others. In other words, this heightened awareness can foster a society where people are not only more understanding of each other but also more willing to act for the greater good.

Healing the Wounds of Community

Beyond individual experiences, psychedelics hold the promise of community healing. Our communities are the bedrock of society, yet they are often fractured by collective trauma - be it historical injustices, or societies grappling with systemic inequalities, or the scars of conflict. Psychedelics hold a unique potential to address these deep-seated wounds and repressed traumas. Picture communities coming together, using these substances in a supportive and guided manner to heal together. The shared experience of psychedelic healing can help address these traumas, facilitating a process of communal healing creating bonds of unity, mutual support, and a renewed sense of purpose. This is not just about individual healing; it's about transforming the very fabric of our communities, fostering resilience, and a collective spirit of recovery.

A New Dawn in Mental Health

For those who have long battled the shadows of PTSD, depression, and anxiety, psychedelics offer a beacon of hope. For too long, conventional treatments for conditions like PTSD, depression, and anxiety have often fallen short, leaving many without relief, and in despair, denying the healing to those who have been underserved by conventional methods.

But psychedelics can revolutionize mental health care, offering profound relief where conventional methods are struggling or have failed. Envision a mental health system that doesn't just treat symptoms but addresses the root causes of suffering with empathy and holistic care. This new approach offers a new paradigm - one that is more holistic and patient-centered. These substances can provide profound therapeutic benefits, helping individuals to process and integrate their experiences in ways that traditional therapies might not. Imagine a mental health care system that embraces these tools, offering hope and even a cure.

The Transformative Ripple Effect

The ripple effect of integrating psychedelics into mainstream society is vast. When individuals experience deep healing and personal growth, they naturally influence those around them.
By reaching into the hearts of both seasoned users and those considering the journey, we can begin to appreciate the profound societal implications of therapeutic psychedelics. journey at a time.

As we examine these broader societal impacts, you are invited to consider the transformative potential of psychedelics beyond the realm of individual therapy. The integration of psychedelics into mainstream medicine and society at large could challenge existing paradigms, encouraging us to adopt more holistic approaches to mental health and well-being.

Exploring these facets, we can begin to envision a world where psychedelics play a key role in fostering a more empathetic and understanding global community. The societal implications of therapeutic psychedelics are vast, offering the promise of deep, systemic change that can benefit us all. These substances offer more than just personal insights; they hold the promise of deep, systemic change that can touch every aspect of our lives. Imagine a world healed, one journey at a time.

FINAL THOUGHTS

As we come to the end of *My Healing Journey with The Golden Teacher*, it is important to reflect on the key points discussed throughout this book, highlighting both the promise and the challenges inherent in therapeutic psychedelic journeys. My story is one of personal transformation, but it is also a testament to the broader implications and potential of psychedelics in the realm of medicine and mental health treatment.

Throughout the chapters, we've endeavoured to explore the deep history of psychedelic use, from ancient and indigenous practices to their modern resurgence amidst scientific scrutiny. We've delved into the legal and ethical landscapes that shape the current and future accessibility of these substances, recognizing the delicate balance between regulation and innovation. The chapter on preparation underscored the importance of set and setting, the role of therapists, and the techniques for integrating insights gained during journeys into everyday life. Practical guidance was provided for potential users, emphasizing safety, consent, and the creation of supportive environments.

The profound personal narratives shared in these pages illustrate the transformative power of psychedelics. They reveal how these substances can facilitate deep healing, particularly for those grappling with trauma and repressed issues. My own journey, masked for years by a relentless focus on work and mundane activities, serves as a beacon of hope for others seeking to break free from their past and achieve lasting healing.

As we look to the future, the potential of psychedelics in holistic treatment cannot be overstated. The therapeutic benefits are vast, but they come with a responsibility to approach these substances with respect and mindfulness. Continued research and responsible practice are essential to unlocking their full potential, ensuring that they can be safely and effectively integrated into therapeutic contexts.

In closing, I advocate for the thoughtful integration of psychedelics into mental health treatment. When used with intention and care, they offer a powerful tool for healing and growth, helping individuals to navigate their traumas and achieve a more enlightened state of being. May this book serve as both a guide and an inspiration, not precluding caution, for those on their own healing journeys, illuminating the path toward a brighter, more self compassionate future.

SUGGESTED FURTHER READING AND RESOURCES

I add here a few of the many highly regarded books on the topic of therapeutic psychedelics and psychedelic journeys that you might find valuable for study. These books offer a comprehensive look at the scientific, therapeutic, historical, and personal aspects of psychedelics. However, dear reader, Care and Caution are advised!

"Trauma is not what happens to you but what happens inside you" - Gabor Maté

"The Myth of Normal: Trauma, Illness and Healing in a Toxic Culture" by Gabor Maté

This book explores trauma and healing in the inimicable style of Gabor Maté defining trauma and providing healing interventions.

"How to Change Your Mind" by Michael Pollan

This book explores the history, science, and therapeutic potential of psychedelics. Pollan provides a detailed account of his own experiences and the current research in the field.

"The Psychedelic Explorer's Guide: Safe, Therapeutic, and Sacred Journeys" by James Fadiman

James Fadiman offers practical advice for safe and effective psychedelic experiences, drawing on decades of research and personal accounts.

"Psychedelic Medicine: The Healing Powers of LSD, MDMA, Psilocybin, and Ayahuasca" by Dr. Richard Louis Miller

This book compiles insights from experts on the therapeutic uses of various psychedelics, discussing their potential to treat mental health issues.

"Acid Test: LSD, Ecstasy, and the Power to Heal" by Tom Shroder

Tom Shroder delves into the history and resurgence of psychedelic research, focusing on the therapeutic applications of LSD and MDMA.

"The Doors of Perception" by Aldous Huxley

Although not a modern guide, Huxley's classic work remains influential in understanding the subjective effects of psychedelics and their potential for expanding consciousness.

"Sacred Knowledge: Psychedelics and Religious Experiences" by William A. Richards

William Richards explores the intersection of psychedelics and spirituality, highlighting their potential to induce profound religious experiences.

"Listening to Ayahuasca: New Hope for Depression, Addiction, PTSD, and Anxiety" by Rachel Harris

This book offers insights into the therapeutic use of ayahuasca, supported by personal stories and clinical research.

"Pihkal: A Chemical Love Story" and "Tihkal: The Continuation" by Alexander and Ann Shulgin

These books provide detailed information on various psychoactive compounds, their synthesis, and their effects, written by renowned chemists and psychonauts.

"The Harvard Psychedelic Club" by Don Lattin

Don Lattin chronicles the lives of four influential figures in the 1960s psychedelic movement and their contributions to the field.

"The Psychedelic Renaissance: Reassessing the Role of Psychedelic Drugs in 21st Century Psychiatry and Society" by Ben Sessa

Ben Sessa reviews the current state of psychedelic research and its potential to revolutionize psychiatry.

"The Little Book of Psychedelic Substances – A Psychedelic Drug Fact Book"

This is a booklet brought out by MAPS for Psychedelic Support for beginners.

Happy exploring…!

REFERENCES

Here are some academic journals that have published significant research on psychedelics over the past decade, and I have drawn from:

Journal of Psychopharmacology
This journal publishes research on the effects of drugs on behavior, including studies on the therapeutic potential of psychedelics like psilocybin, LSD, and MDMA.

Frontiers in Psychology
This open-access journal features articles on a wide range of psychological topics, including numerous studies on psychedelic therapy and its effects on mental health.

Drug and Alcohol Dependence
This journal focuses on the biomedical and psychosocial aspects of substance use and addiction, often publishing research on the use of psychedelics in treating addiction.

Psychopharmacology
A leading journal in the field, it covers the effects of drugs on mood, behavior, and cognition, with many

studies on psychedelic substances.

Journal of Clinical Psychopharmacology

This journal provides clinical research on psychopharmacology, including the therapeutic use of psychedelics in mental health treatment.

The American Journal of Psychiatry

As a premier journal in the field of psychiatry, it has published influential research on the potential of psychedelics to treat psychiatric disorders.

International Journal of Neuropsychopharmacology

This journal includes research on the effects of drugs on the nervous system, including studies on the neurobiological mechanisms of psychedelics.

The Lancet Psychiatry

A leading journal that covers various aspects of mental health and psychiatry, including high-impact studies on the therapeutic use of psychedelics.

PLoS ONE

An open-access journal that publishes research across all scientific disciplines, including numerous studies on the therapeutic applications of psychedelics.

Neuropharmacology

This journal focuses on the effects of drugs on

the nervous system and brain function, including research on the neuropharmacology of psychedelics.

These journals have contributed significantly to the body of research on psychedelics, covering a wide range of topics from clinical trials and therapeutic applications to neurobiological mechanisms and societal impacts.

GLOSSARY OF TERMS

There may be more terms here than in the book but relevant to our topic.

5-HT2A Receptors
A subtype of serotonin receptors in the brain that psychedelics primarily bind to, leading to altered states of consciousness.

Ambient Music
Soft, calming music used to create a soothing atmosphere during a psychedelic session, aiding in relaxation and immersion.

Ancient and Indigenous Practices
Historical and cultural uses of psychedelics for spiritual, healing, and ceremonial purposes by various cultures around the world.

Awakening a Compassionate Society
The concept of using psychedelics to foster a more empathetic and understanding society by helping individuals recognize the interconnectedness of all life and transcend personal struggles to foster

kindness and well-being for others.

Ayahuasca
A potent psychoactive brew made from the Banisteriopsis caapi vine and other ingredients, used traditionally by Amazonian tribes for spiritual and healing purposes.

Bad Trip
A negative or frightening psychedelic experience, often due to lack of preparation or support, characterized by anxiety, paranoia, or distress.

Beckley Foundation
A think tank and NGO that initiates, directs, and supports research into the benefits and mechanisms of psychedelics and cannabis.

Blissful State
A state of profound happiness and contentment often reached during a psychedelic journey, characterized by feelings of joy and interconnectedness.

Boundless Curiosity
An open and inquisitive mindset often experienced during a psychedelic journey, encouraging exploration and acceptance of the unknown.

Breakthrough Therapy Designation

A status granted by the FDA to expedite the development and review of drugs that show substantial improvement over existing treatments for serious conditions.

Catharsis

The process of releasing and thereby providing relief from strong or repressed emotions, often experienced during a psychedelic session.

Client-Centric Perspectives

The approach in therapy that emphasizes the client's experiences, needs, and perspectives as central to the therapeutic process.

Clinical Trials

Research studies conducted to evaluate the safety and efficacy of medical interventions, including psychedelics, in treating various conditions.

Cognitive Loop

A repetitive cycle of distressing thoughts or feelings, often triggered during challenging psychedelic experiences and difficult to break without guidance.

Collective Trauma

Psychological and emotional damage experienced by a group of people due to shared traumatic events, such as war, systemic racism, or natural disasters.

Community Healing
The potential of psychedelics to address and heal collective traumas within communities, such as historical injustices and systemic inequalities, by facilitating shared healing experiences.

Confidentiality
The ethical and legal duty of therapists to protect the privacy of their clients and keep their personal information secure.

Consent
The voluntary agreement to participate in psychedelic therapy, with full understanding of the risks, benefits, and nature of the treatment.

Contraindications
Specific conditions or factors that increase the risks associated with a particular treatment, making it unsuitable for certain individuals.

Countercultural Movement
A social movement in the 1960s that rejected mainstream norms and values, often embracing psychedelic substances for personal and societal transformation.

Cultural Sensitivity
Awareness and respect for the cultural background and beliefs of clients, incorporating culturally

appropriate practices into therapy.

Default Mode Network (DMN)
A brain network associated with self-referential thoughts and the ego, which psychedelics can disrupt, leading to a sense of interconnectedness and reduced ego.

Decriminalization
The reduction or elimination of criminal penalties for certain acts, such as the possession and use of psychedelics, while keeping them illegal.

Debriefing
A post-session discussion between the therapist and the individual to review and process the experiences and emotions encountered during the psychedelic journey.

Debriefing Sessions
Post-session meetings where clients process and integrate their psychedelic experiences.

Dendritic Growth
The growth of dendrites (branches of neurons), which can be enhanced by psychedelics, leading to increased brain connectivity.

Ego Dissolution
A profound experience during which a user loses the

sense of individual self, often leading to spiritual or existential insights in therapeutic settings.

Eleusinian Mysteries

Ancient Greek religious rites held in Eleusis, involving the consumption of a psychoactive potion called kykeon, which facilitated profound spiritual experiences of death and rebirth.

Emotional Rigidity

Fixed or suppressed emotional responses that therapeutic psychedelics may help release, fostering emotional healing.

Empathy

The ability to understand and share the feelings of another, which can be enhanced through psychedelic experiences.

Enlightened State of Being

A heightened state of awareness and understanding, often achieved through deep personal and spiritual insights gained from psychedelic experiences.

Enlightenment

A state of heightened awareness and understanding, often associated with spiritual awakening and profound insights into oneself and the nature of reality.

Epiphanies
Sudden, profound realizations or insights that
significantly alter an individual's understanding or
perspective.

Eye Mask
A mask worn over the eyes to block out visual
stimuli, helping individuals focus inward during a
psychedelic session.

Flashbacks
Recurrent, often unexpected, re-experiencing of
aspects of a past psychedelic experience, which can
occur in HPPD or as residual effects.

Golden Teacher
A popular strain of psilocybin mushrooms known
for its golden caps and spiritual and insightful
experiences often reported by users.

Hallucinations
Sensory experiences without actual external stimuli,
commonly visual or auditory, that psychedelics can
induce in varying intensity.

Healing
The process of recovering from physical, emotional,
or psychological trauma, leading to a state of
improved well-being and health.

Holistic Care

A comprehensive approach to health care that addresses the physical, emotional, social, and spiritual needs of individuals.

Holistic Treatment

An approach to therapy that considers the whole person, including their physical, mental, emotional, and spiritual well-being.

HPPD

(Hallucinogen Persisting Perception Disorder)
A condition where users experience flashbacks or residual sensory disturbances long after psychedelic use.

Integration

The process of understanding and assimilating the insights from a psychedelic experience, often facilitated by therapy to enhance benefits and minimize risks.

Imperial College London

An academic institution conducting significant research into the effects of psychedelics on the brain and mental health.

Informed Consent

The process by which a patient is fully informed about the potential risks, benefits, and uncertainties of a treatment before agreeing to participate.

Initial Consultation

The first meeting between a client and therapist to discuss the client's mental health history, current psychological state, and therapeutic goals.

Inner Peace

A state of mental and emotional calmness and stability, free from stress, anxiety, and inner turmoil.

Inner Shadows

The repressed fears, insecurities, and unresolved emotions within an individual, often confronted during a psychedelic journey.

Integration

The process of incorporating insights and experiences from a psychedelic journey into one's everyday life to promote long-term healing and personal growth.

Integration Protocols

Structured approaches to help clients incorporate insights gained from psychedelic experiences into their daily lives.

Interconnectedness

The recognition of the interdependence of all living beings, often a profound insight gained through psychedelic experiences.

Journaling

The practice of writing down thoughts, emotions, and insights during or after a psychedelic experience to aid in reflection and integration.

Johns Hopkins University

An academic institution known for its pioneering research into the therapeutic potential of psilocybin.

Kykeon

A psychoactive potion used in the Eleusinian Mysteries, believed to induce profound spiritual experiences.

Lemon-Ginger Tea

A herbal tea preparation often used to mix with psilocybin powder, enhancing the absorption and mitigating nausea during a psychedelic session.

LSD (Lysergic Acid Diethylamide)

A powerful synthetic hallucinogen that causes significant changes in perception, sometimes leading to altered states of consciousness.

Mazatec People

An indigenous group from Oaxaca, Mexico, known for their traditional use of psilocybin mushrooms in spiritual and healing ceremonies.

Measure 109
An initiative passed in Oregon allowing the
regulated medical use of psilocybin for mental
health treatment.

Mental Health System
The network of services, institutions, and
professionals that provide mental health care and
support.

MDMA
(3,4-Methylenedioxymethamphetamine)
Also known as "ecstasy," a synthetic psychoactive
drug that induces feelings of euphoria, emotional
openness, and empathy, altering mood and
perception, known for its potential use in therapy
for PTSD and other conditions.

**Multidisciplinary Association for Psychedelic
Studies (MAPS)**
A research and educational organization that
develops medical, legal, and cultural contexts
for people to benefit from the careful uses of
psychedelics and marijuana.

Neuroplasticity
The brain's ability to reorganize itself by forming
new neural connections throughout life, often
enhanced by psychedelics in therapeutic contexts to

aid in trauma processing.

Paranoia
Intense feelings of suspicion or fear, sometimes experienced during psychedelic use, especially in recreational settings without support.

Patient-Centered Care
A health care approach that respects and responds to the preferences, needs, and values of patients, ensuring that patient values guide all clinical decisions.

Peer Support Groups
Groups of individuals with shared experiences who provide mutual support and understanding.

Personal Narratives
Stories and experiences shared by individuals, offering insights and reflections on their journeys, particularly in the context of therapeutic psychedelics.

Personal Transformation
Significant and lasting change in an individual's behavior, perspective, and emotional state, often as a result of psychedelic therapy.

Psilocybin
A naturally occurring psychedelic compound found

in certain mushrooms, used both recreationally
and therapeutically for its mood-enhancing and
consciousness-expanding effects.

Psychedelics
Substances like psilocybin, LSD, and MDMA that alter
perception, mood, and thought processes, often used
either for therapeutic or recreational purposes.

Psychedelic Healing
The process of using psychedelic substances to
facilitate emotional and psychological healing.

Psychedelic Renaissance
The current resurgence of scientific and public
interest in the therapeutic potential of psychedelics,
driven by new research and advocacy.

Psychedelic Science Funders Collaborative
An organization that funds and supports
scientific research on the therapeutic potential of
psychedelics.

Psychedelic Therapy
A therapeutic practice involving the controlled use
of psychedelic substances to facilitate emotional and
psychological healing and growth.

Random Blood Glucose
A measurement of blood sugar levels, checked before

a psychedelic session to ensure the individual is within healthy parameters.

Recreational Use
The unsupervised consumption of psychedelics for enjoyment, mood enhancement, or curiosity, often in uncontrolled settings.

Regulated Dosing
The controlled administration of a specific amount of a psychedelic substance, typically within a clinical setting.

Revolution in Mental Health Care
The transformative potential of psychedelics to radically change the way mental health conditions are treated, moving towards more effective and holistic approaches.

Self-Compassion
Treating oneself with kindness and understanding, particularly when confronting inner pain and suffering during and after a psychedelic experience.

Self-Discovery
The process of gaining a deeper understanding of oneself, including one's beliefs, desires, and motivations, often achieved through introspection and therapy.

Serotonin System/Serotonergic System
The neural pathways in the brain involving
serotonin, a neurotransmitter significantly
impacted by psychedelics, influencing mood,
cognition, and perception,

Sessions
Individual instances of therapeutic experiences,
often involving the use of psychedelics, where
specific goals and outcomes are pursued.

Set and Setting
A concept emphasizing the importance of mental
state (set) and the physical and social environment
(setting) in which a psychedelic experience takes
place, both of which significantly influence and
shape psychedelic experiences.

Shared Experience
The collective participation in an event or activity,
which can strengthen bonds and foster a sense of
community, especially in therapeutic settings.

Shamanic Rituals
Ceremonial practices conducted by shamans, who
are believed to interact with the spiritual world and
use various substances, including psychedelics, to
induce altered states of consciousness for healing
and divination.

Soma

A sacred brew mentioned in ancient Vedic texts, used in spiritual rituals to achieve divine communion, possibly derived from the Ephedra plant or other psychoactive ingredients.

Subconscious

The part of the mind that holds thoughts, memories, and desires not currently in conscious awareness but which influence behavior and emotions.

Supportive Environment

A safe and nurturing setting provided by therapists and guides during psychedelic therapy to ensure a positive and therapeutic experience.

Support System

The network of professional or personal support essential for safe, effective therapeutic psychedelic use, helping users process intense experiences.

Synaptic Plasticity

The ability of synapses (connections between neurons) to strengthen or weaken over time, influenced by psychedelic substances to promote new neural connections.

Systemic Change

Fundamental and comprehensive changes to systems or institutions, often driven by the integration of new practices or paradigms.

Therapeutic Alliance
The relationship between a therapist and client, characterized by trust, empathy, and mutual respect.

Therapeutic Benefits
The positive effects of psychedelics in treating mental health conditions and promoting psychological well-being.

Therapeutic Contexts
Settings and conditions under which psychedelic therapy is conducted, emphasizing safety, professionalism, and ethical practices.

Therapeutic Intent
A clear, focused goal established before a therapeutic psychedelic session, guiding the experience to maximize potential mental health benefits.

Therapeutic Process
The structured approach to treatment that includes preparation, the therapeutic experience itself, and post-experience integration to facilitate healing.

Therapeutic Use
The supervised, intentional administration of psychedelics under professional guidance to treat mental health issues like depression or PTSD.

Therapist
A trained professional who guides and supports individuals through their psychedelic experiences, ensuring safety and facilitating emotional and psychological breakthroughs.

Therapist/Healer
A trained professional who guides and supports individuals through therapeutic processes, including psychedelic therapy, ensuring safety and facilitating healing.

Therapy Dog
A specially trained dog that provides comfort and support during therapeutic sessions, aiding in the emotional and psychological healing process.

Trauma
A deeply distressing or disturbing experience, often the focus of healing in psychedelic therapy.

Traumatic Re-emergence
The resurfacing of past traumatic memories and emotions during a psychedelic journey, often leading to catharsis and healing.

Transformative Potential
The ability of psychedelic experiences to bring about significant personal growth, healing, and changes in

perspective.

Transformation
A profound change in an individual's mental, emotional, or spiritual state, often resulting from therapeutic or life-changing experiences.

Transcendence
The experience of going beyond ordinary limits, often described in psychedelic experiences as a sense of unity with the universe or a higher state of consciousness.

Unity
A state of being united or joined as a whole, often a profound insight gained through psychedelic experiences that emphasize the interconnectedness of all life.

Vedic Hindu Rituals
Ancient spiritual practices from the Indian subcontinent, as mentioned in the Rigveda, that included the use of a sacred brew called Soma, believed to induce divine experiences.

Vivid Imagery
Intensely clear and colorful visual experiences often encountered during a psychedelic journey, contributing to the profound nature of the session.

War on Drugs
A campaign initiated by President Richard Nixon
in the early 1970s to reduce illegal drug use, which
led to the prohibition and stigmatization of many
substances, including psychedelics.

Well-Being
A state of being comfortable, healthy, or happy,
which psychedelics can enhance by helping
individuals process and integrate their experiences.

ABOUT THE AUTHOR

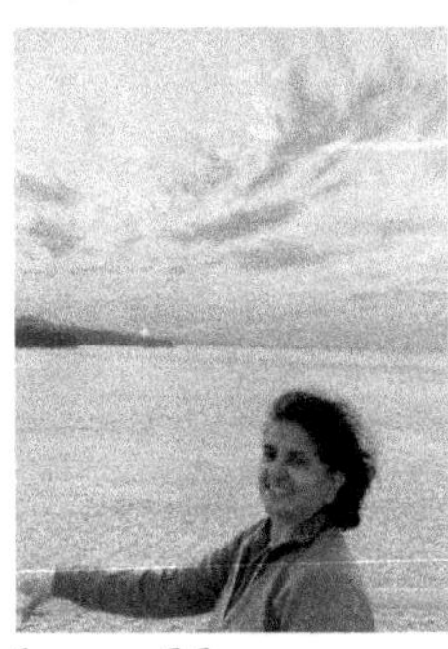 Vidya Shastry is a seasoned healthcare professional with a diverse background in nursing, clinical research, and mental health. With a Master of Science in Cell Biology and advanced qualifications in practical nursing and foot care, Vidya Shastry has honed her expertise across various domains, including geriatrics, forensic rehabilitation, and trauma-informed care. Her extensive experience spans over two decades, where she has contributed significantly to patient care in both in-patient and out-patient settings, and as an educator, shaping the next generation of nurses. Her commitment to continuous learning and development has equipped her with a unique perspective on the intersection of traditional and alternative therapeutic approaches.

As an author, Vidya Shastry draws upon her rich professional journey and personal encounters with mental illness and rehabilitation. Her book, "Awakening and Healing with the Golden Teacher:

A Transformative Journey with Psilocybin," reflects her deep understanding of trauma-informed care and the challenges faced in balancing state-approved pharmaceuticals with emerging psychedelic therapies. Through this work, she offers a compelling narrative that advocates for a broader, more integrative approach to mental health treatment, underscoring the potential of psilocybin in fostering healing and personal transformation.

www.ingramcontent.com/pod-product-compliance
Lightning Source LLC
Chambersburg PA
CBHW051750250726
48659CB00001B/348